NOURISHMENT FOR A SOUND LIFE

Live A Healthy Life With The Right Food

By Raymond Armstrong

Table of content

Foreword

Simply said, the body's two distinct and intricate processes for generating energy are significantly different from one another. Since energy is essential to the human action and survival very existence the dual energy style are mutually supportive of one another. This book demonstrates meals that are most energy-boosting.

We decide to continue a healthy lifestyle since it happens so regularly and exercise program with enthusiasm and perhaps much fanfare but in the first week of implementing the plan,Everything comes to a stop. Why do we fail to maintain the diet?

strategies, such as the early-morning jog routines and exercise schedules that we produce?What can we do, for our own sakes as well as the sakes of others who depend on us, to ensure that we continue with our plans?

Do you eat merely to sate your hunger or to enhance your joyful taste buds? Or do you consume to gain more control over who you are? This eBook demonstrates how you can improve your life.

merely by ensuring that you eat will make things far more ideal.

Introduction

The essential and first to be utilized energy framework is the vigorous framework. This framework involves oxygen for the capability of the muscles what's more, requests a considerable amount from the general body framework.

This request generally expands the rate and profundity of relaxing

furthermore, blood supply principally in light of the relating increment of the pulse. At the point when the body requires more energy, which can't be met

because of the raised requirement for more oxygen then the body framework consequently changed to the anaerobic energy framework.

This framework can deliver energy without the need to utilize oxygen.

This energy is produced through the reasonable or right utilization of food varieties. The food varieties devoured direct the sorts of energy levels everybody can deliver.

Muscle weakness typically happens when all the energy sources are depleted which can be credited to different reasons; the most convincing one

relies especially upon the sorts of food varieties ate.

There are a few classes of food varieties that produce different valuable components for the human body framework and noticing the ones that make or upgrade the energy creating sources is valuable to be aware. Hence, this information ought to help the individual pick the right kinds of food sources.

The high-impact framework works by separating the carbs, unsaturated fats and amino acids in the food varieties devoured while the anaerobic framework lets energy out of the food varieties put away in the body, generally during extraordinary action sessions. Assuming we catch wind of the disappointment of diets or rec center plans surrounding us, generally it isn'ttheir issue.

Usually the issue of the people began with much upheaval about going through these plans, leaving out nothing their associates and colleagues about it, and afterward didn't keep those projects. The people who leave the exercise or abstain from food midway don't see the benefits, normally, furthermore, everyone faults the arrangement.

What the world necessities these days is certainly not a new wellbeing or wellness program or an eating regimen, however it requires inspiration.

It needs the right kind of mentality to completely finish whatever arrangement they have decided as far as possible.In the event that they can do that, the greater part of the medical problems that are connected with way of life circumstances will become outdated. What's more, we don't have

to visit the edges of the earth to find this inspiration. The inspiration lies here, inside us; we basically have to look through it out and use it.

One age back, people wouldn't fantasy about getting anything low quality food they might set up to take care of their countenances.

These days, that's what we do so nonchalantly. "I'm ravenous" generally signifies "I need a burger or a frank, logical with chips on the side and some cola." And, "I'm on a tight eating routine" signifies "I'm on an artificially ridden pill which will overcome my craving and deny my assortment of nutrients." It's really no big surprise that we are confronting so many medical problems today.

Our wellbeing is a mark of what we consume. The sorry condition that we're living in is certainly not a singular issue; it's a worldwide issue. The world is eating inaccurately. Six in each ten people in the US is overweight, and the number is going to

be eight in each ten people when we hit 2021.

Is it safe to say that we are genuinely pondering this? We aren't. Indeed, even as you're concentrating on this eBook, you probably have a bundle of chips on the side. Do you have at least some idea that what you spent on that bundle, which is filling your stomach with the absolute most poisonous synthetic substances known to humankind, could rather have taken care of a thin youth in Ruanda?

However, it's not just about being magnanimous. It's about ourselves as well. Indeed, we must be egotistical. With such horrifying wellbeing figures, would we confirm or deny that we are setting out toward destruction? We're certainly not eating right. Whatever overabundance stuff that brings - stoutness also, the different medical affliction afterward - we must be ready for it.

So the following time you see that a program has fizzled or is getting a ton of analysis, recall that the analysis isn't likely in light of the fact that the program remains in peril. In most cases, it is on the grounds that individuals started with extraordinary aims and afterward didn't follow the program as they ought to have.

Chapter1 The manner in which you contemplate food

Your believe

We have wandered terribly with our dietary patterns hitherto.Except if we check out the situation and take matters in our own hands, matters won't improve.

The number 1 thing is mindfulness. We need to realize what food varieties are right for ourselves and what are not. We need to go back to preparing and grasp what the supplements are that your body genuinely needs and in what sum.

Then, at that point, we need to fabricate a dietary routine for us and our friends and family with the goal that we eat better. We need to cut down on every one of the food varieties that are unfriendly - the sugars, the fats,the starches, we don't genuinely need them - and consolidate food sources that might support our wellbeing.

This sounds excessively sermonizing, I get it. In any case, that is the just respite we have. Assuming we chomp on Oreos, we're never going to improve. In any case, there's trust.

Trust lies in the way that there are a great deal of food sources out there that are essentially pretty much as scrumptious as those terrible unhealthy foods yet we have hardly any insight into them.

These are the food varieties that we have hardly any familiarity with yet, we likely could do without them or as we don't have the foggiest idea how to fix them, yet a solid cookbook might help you in understanding grouped fascinating approaches to sound cooking. Indeed, even with a similar sort

of diet you eat, you can invoke some delectable sound dishes. Indeed, it's all a lot of conceivable. You can change your dietary patterns to a major degree, while at a similar time taking care of your sense of taste.The truth of the matter is that the weight reduction industry is capable in a critical way towards this ruin of the created human race. They should continue to sell their Atkins' and Jenny

Craigs and Zones and Medi-quick and hence the

media never lets you know how we might take things in your own hands.

They show us stylish before-after photos of an individual with a foot-long sub and afterward similar person with 6 pack abs and tell us that the eating regimen made that conceivable.

Notwithstanding,the truth of the mater is, if we were to get our head together, we may handily do that as well, without burning through 1000s of dollars on those who consumes less calories. Also, what do we need to do?

2 essential things: - Control what we consume. Enjoy actual effort.

Presently, is that an excessive amount to achieve? Don't we owe that to our body that has served us so well such a long time? Don't we owe that to ourselves and our family?

Chapter2 whole grains and honey

A Honey's inherent advantages have long been understood and respected. In addition to its fantastic flavor, honey is a natural supply of carbohydrates, a fuel for boosting energy performance, stamina, and a reduction in the intensity of muscular exhaustion.This is particularly helpful for competitors. The sugar content in the honey assists with assuming a part in forestalling weakness during exercise meetings and furthermore during instructional courses for sports aficionado.These sugars make ups are separated into glucose and fructose also, capabilities in various however praising ways. The glucose content in the honey is for the most part consumed at a quicker rate and radiates a prompt jolt of energy while the fructose works at a more slow speed for a more supportable and delayed energy payment.With regards to tending to glucose levels in the body framework, honey has been known to assist with keeping the levels steady.

As honey is a charming food item and it's normal in its structure,consuming it's anything but an undeniably challenging activity. Individuals, everything being equal, are by and large very able to consume honey in any of its going with structures. It's even famous with youngsters.

The energy delivered from consuming a modest quantity of honey day to day assists youngsters with adapting to the actual types of day to day school exercises and sports responsibilities.

For the grown-ups too consuming an everyday little portion of honey can go quite far in keeping the energy levels at its best during a requesting day at work. Making sandwiches with honey went with different fillings is one approach to making a

wonderful tidbit.Applying honey on a newly toasted cut of bread is likewise a welcome breakfast elective. Adding honey to drinks all things being equal of utilizing sugar is empowered. The vast majority today need a speedy fix for their energy helping requirements and this typically comes in the unfortunate types of sports beverages, espresso and refined carbs like sugar and keeping in mind that bread.

However these produce the ideal elevated energy levels, it ought to be noticed that this energy is genuinely brief and the sluggishness that follows is generally more intensely felt. In this manner
selecting to consume some type of entire grains isn't just a better other option but at the same time is a lot better.Entire grains give the energy that arrives in a more mind boggling structure what separates over a more extended timeframe. This then
makes the stage for supporting the energy levels for longer periods.

Due to its more complicated make up the entire grains come with a variety of valuable components like minerals, nutrients,phytonutrients, and fiber which are likewise wealthy in fiber. Adding
the entire grain fixings is any dish frequently finishes the flavor or upgrades it out and out. Entire grains can the different
structures like wheat, oat, grain, maize, earthy colored rice, faro, spelt,emmer, einkorn, rye, millet, buckwheat, and some more.

These can then be made into different items like entirety wheat flour, entire wheat bread, entire wheat pasta, rolled oats or oat groats, triticale flour, popcorn and teff flour.

The advantages of consuming entire grains reliably can help decline the gamble of coronary illness, lower cholesterol levels safeguard against many sorts of malignant growth and aid weight the board. Entire grains ought not be mistaken for its lesser and more refined "cousin". However refined grains have a few advantages it is in every case better to settle overall grain options.

Chapter3 Good Oils And Proteins

It is now widely known that nuts significantly aid in keeping many illnesses under control or preventing them altogether.For example, nuts have been known to have the option to keep the

probability of coronary heart infections showing, in any event, for those entire come from a long queue of relatives with this issue.

Consuming nuts like almonds and pecans have been known to lower serum cholesterol focuses inside the body framework.

Nuts are additionally enthusiastically suggested for those people experiencing insulin obstruction issues like diabetics.

Going to nuts rather that low quality food to control desires is too another better other option. Containing fundamental unsaturated fats is

likewise one more in addition to moment that it comes to picking nuts as a better other option.

Since nuts are sound and can be consumed in its crude structure, it is additionally one more added benefit to keeping these around and convenient as bites.

Almonds are frequently used to standardize blood lipids due to their gradual process attributes, which help to keep the blood sugar levels reliably sound. Rich in a differed measure of various supplements the almond is a famous added substance to the lifeless diet of most Mediterranean individuals.

The Brazil nut is additionally another nutritious nut which accompanies its own arrangement of advantages when consumed with some restraint. Noted for its omega 3 unsaturated fat substance, the Brazil nut is likewise a decent wellspring of calcium.Cashew nut is another exceptionally well known nut that is frequently consumed as a salted bite. Anyway it would be a lot better food

item without the expansion of salt, as it is now very much a delightful nut all alone. In certain areas of the planet these nuts are made into oils.

The choice cycle ought to be finished with a little information as contingent exclusively upon what the unaided eye sees isn't enough.

For the most part lean meats got from hamburger cuts ought to incorporate round, throw, sirloin and tenderloin, while the cuts

from pork or sheep would comprise tenderloin, midsection hacks and leg.

The least fatty pieces of the poultry would be the bosom region without the skin.

However there are many reasons individuals kill meat from their everyday eating routine, there is no proof to show that this is a decent or on the other hand awful decision not would it be advisable for it be trailed by all.

Anyway the significant highlight note here is the decision of the sorts of meats that would make the utilization sound and this would commonly mean meats with lesser measure of fat content. However white meat is in no way, shape or form ailing in fat content, it is by examination significantly less in fat substance than red meats. The dietary benefit of consuming lean meats is very broad and adjusted.Lean meats have a by and large higher and cleaner content of protein which is a vital contributing component to principal primary and utilitarian advancement of each and every cell

food and arrangement.

Lean meats are likewise a decent wellspring of fundamental amino acids especially sulfur amino acids. When contrasted with the stomach related rates the proteins in meats work quicker than the one contained in the beans and entire wheat range.

Lean meat is likewise a decent wellspring of iron. Since lack of iron is moderate it is frequently not identified until a later stage where sickliness has created.

Chapter4 The Advantages

Your health improves

Even if we had a library full of literature on the benefits of healthy diet, they wouldn't fully address what benefits are actually present. The most crucial advantage you develop control over your weight.

By eating properly, you also ensure that your metabolic processes, particularly those of your immune system and keep your digestive system functioning properly.You're also protected from a variety of chronic disorders, starting

from cardiovascular conditions including elevated blood pressure and coronary artery hypertension and diabetes.

More economically sound spend substantially less money when you eat healthfully. Your grocery expenses drop significantly, yet you don't see a sudden spike if credit card debt is already a problem, farther into it.Additionally, you save a ton of money on all the healthcare costs you'd incur if a problem arises as a result of your eating disorders.

Your body contains less toxins.

Nowadays, a lot of foods are poisonous because of the synthetic substances that they contain. If you're trying to eat correctly, you have a considerably lower chance of ingesting these pollutants.
One of the fundamental tenets of eating healthfully is that you should not consume any artificial food.
Additionally, you'll be able to cut back on vices like drunkenness and smoking. A beer nearly always signifies a night out with the guys. When you eat less will make you less interested in the beer. Likewise, you won't want the one (or more) required cigarettes that you typically smoke following every meal.

A more active lifestyle

You'll discover that you can function much more effectively when you eat better. You have more time to workout,increase your work, play, and travel to increase your
increased productivity in life.

That sure beats being a slob and relaxing on the couch while you're obese.

Couch the entire day, is that right? You have the capacity to do more.

Being involved with your loved ones and friends, that's for sure makes your life richer.

Optimal Social Life

Forget about the "fat fetishism," overweight people don't look good. There is a severe societal stigma surrounding

excess bodily weight in the incorrect locations.Your excess weight could actually interfere with a partner. Not merely

example, those people whose eating habits are out of control and who consequently society despises their weight and views them as being

people with uncontrollable primal impulses.This kind of psychology does exist, but very few people have it.

When you eat healthfully, you'll learn that

Such problems vanish.

A Conclusion

There are several well-liked diets available today, but the majority of them are harmful and occasionally even dangerous. This will clarify how to maintain a lifelong healthy diet and away from poor eating habits.

Calculate the amount of calories your body needs to operate every day.

The range of this figure depends on your metabolism and your level of physical activity. Depending on the type of
someone who gains ten pounds after smelling a piece of pizza, your daily calorie consumption should remain the equivalent of 1500 calories for women and 2000 calories for men.
Additionally, your body mass affects this: For naturally bigger people, more calories are recommended, and for smaller people, fewer calories. If you're the type of person who enjoys food or haven't gained any weight, you might want to consume 1000–2000 more calories per day,
somewhat less for females.

Avoid greasy foods.

For your body to function properly, you must consume fat from food. But it's important to choose the right kinds of fats:
The majority of vegetable oils and animal fats are high in the type of fatty acids that increase LDL cholesterol; bad cholesterol.
Contrary to popular opinion, consuming cholesterol inevitably build up your body's cholesterol levels.Your body will flush out additional waste if you give it the right resources.These are monounsaturated tools.
unsaturated fats, which you should attempt to routinely consume. Food sources that are wealthy in monounsaturated unsaturated fats are olive oil, nuts, fish oil, and grouped seed oils.

Eat a lot of the right carbs.

You need to eat food sources high in carbs since they're your body's boss wellspring of energy.
Try to select the right carbs.Basic carbs like sugar and refined flour are immediately ingested by the body's gastrointestinal framework.

This incites a kind of carb over-burden, and your body discharges huge measures of insulin to fight the over-burden. Not exclusively is the
abundance insulin awful on your heart, but it supports weight acquire.Eat a lot of carbs, however consume carbs that are gradually processed
by the body, for example, entire grain flour, veggies, oats, and natural grains.

Eat greater feasts from the get-go in the day.

Your digestion decelerates close to the furthest limit of the night
what's more, is less proficient at processing food sources. That implies a greater amount of the
power put away in the food will be stacked away as fat and your
body will not retain as numerous supplements from the feast.
Have a go at eating a medium-sized feast for breakfast, a major dinner for
lunch, and a little feast for supper. Even better, endeavor
consuming 4-6 little feasts over the run of your day.

Give yourself a cheat feast.

Cheating doesn't mean pigging out on every one of some unacceptable food varieties once a
week; it suggests partaking in a food you really love one time each week.
Several cuts of pizza on Sundays, or an enormous cut of
twofold chocolate cake on Saturdays.
This cheat feast will assist you with staying with the adjustment of diet, and
in a couple of ways it's truly great for your body. Extraordinary events,
like birthday events in the family, consider cheat feasts.Get the propensity for eating gradually.
It will fulfill you with less calories and will prevent indulging and heftiness with every one of its ramifications.

Drink a lot of H2O.

It causes you to feel more conscious and empowered, does ponders for your skin and causes you to feel more full so you end up eating less!
Chopping down pop and supplanting it with water will do ponders for you.